Stuttering

Overcome It Quickly In 7 Simple Steps

ARLO MASON

DEDICATION

My family of stutterers, old and new.

CONTENTS

ACKNOWLEDGMENTS

Thank you to
Jerry Morgan and all students of our masterclasses both past and present.

INTRODUCTION

If you struggle with speech because of stuttering, or your child, your ward or your student is the one that has to struggle, it won't be really necessary to tell you what the definition of stuttering is. You already know that the problem is with the first sound of a word. There is no way a person can say the first sound of a word and won't be able to say the entire word no matter how many syllables the word has.

That is exactly what we are going to do for you in 7 steps with this guide. Whether it is stuttering in adults or in kids, or whether you are helping a loved one to find his voice, our guide will make it very easy for you and it will take just a short time to do it.

We will help you identify what makes you stutter. You will learn the factors that worsens the situation and how to overcome them. This guide also covers other matters such as lisping and some common consonant omissions when talking.

Our guide is very simple and the most friendly you can find anywhere. You will find no specialist language that will confuse you or make you feel that the matter is harder than you thought. We use day to day thoughts and ideas to help you grasp the lesson quite easily. And we did our best to use causal and household language as well as to simplify all activities so that anyone can buoy along comfortably.

Many people say that stuttering cannot be stopped because it is in the gene. We are going to surprise you. And trust me, that is not going to be more than 30 days if you put up a hard effort to follow our instructions. For years, we have been doing it. We are never afraid of the gene.

What's in your gene? Did you remember how the Wright Brothers defiled the gravity in the early 20th century?

Unfortunately, most of you have been told in your stuttering groups and communities not to listen to guide information on overcoming the problem. They say that you should just take yourself as you are. Learn self-esteem instead of worrying yourself. You will get frustrated if you try to think that you can get over stuttering. That there is nothing wrong with you.

But who says that something is wrong with you? We have never said that, because our years of helping stutterers with this issue prove the fact. If a person stutters, it doesn't mean that his organs of speech are faulty. We always find that they are working fine. Controlling those organs to say the first sound of the word is at the root of the problem. This is because the ability to do so is allowed to go away too far. When you can't say the sound, you stop. Then, you fight again and again to say it before you get it right It is that control. And you know, as this goes on over a period of time, other habits develop that might not look too appealing.

But don't worry, we are going to help you identify all of that and teach you how you can totally conquer them.

When we say that there is nothing wrong with a stutterer and that his organs of speech have no problem too, we are also actually saying that this is within the scope of the kind of stammer that we handle.

At this point, we would like to mention that we handle only normal stammer. We will talk about that a little bit later. We have nothing to do with stammer that are connected with nervous issues such as muscular dystrophy, sclerosis, Parkinson's and the likes. But those that are hereditary or acquired are all within the ability of our course or guide.

Before we take a short look at the kinds of stuttering, permit me to move back the hands of the clock a little bit. I said earlier that your communities and foundations are afraid of the gene. They think that stammer is hereditary and so, it can never go away. But our own masterclass doesn't have any fear of the gene. We are the owners of Stuttering Help And Solution. We defiled the gene the way the Wright Brothers did gravity by the first airplane.

1
OVERWRITING HEREDITY

I asked what the gene is before. Well all the characters that we inherited through the genes of our parents can be likened to default programs settings of applications running on a computer or mobile. But they are flexible and they can be customized to what you want. I'm going to prove that point. And trust me, all my arguments have been proven by science.

(1) Heredity plays only a small part in human intelligence. A brain-active person gets more connections or synapses in the brain than a brain-lazy individual. And the more connections you develop in your brain, the more intelligent you are.

(2) Heredity has very little control over how our characters are molded. Environment shapes what persons we actually turn out to be in life. For example, identical twins have exactly the same makeup at birth. But if they are separated and raised in different territories, they also get customized differently as they grow up.

(3) Needless to mention how people can even customize their physical attributes these days. We know how athletes and body builders grow their muscles. We are aware of the technologies and techniques of growing boobs and asses.

The list is endless and science has proved all of this. Man has been defiling heredity. So, you will learn how we are going to help you find your voice by challenging and winning the gene.

Now, there is this African proverb that I love so much. "The white man's mind that hatched the idea of the lead in a pencil is the same one that did the eraser." I love it. The proverb is actually saying that the reversal of some realities is through the same process of creating the realities.

That is exactly how our brain works. New habits are formed through creation of new synapses in the brain. Old habits are erased through creation of new counter brain connections. It is all the same process. Everything we do is like that. You keep getting new connections once you make your brain active. If you are always reading or studying to learn something; if you have that kind of strong personal discipline, you will always create new connections for those interests that matter most to you. And if you need to overcome a habit and you have a very strong personal discipline for it and your brain is active for it, you will get new connections that will overshadow the undesirable habit. That is how our brain works. It is always getting new things and it is always writing over something if we are really disciplined for it.

So what will you need for this program? Very few simple things. Before we get to that, I remember I wanted to talk a little bit about normal stuttering and the other type of stuttering.

2
WHEN STUTTERING IS NORMAL OR NOT

This classification is our own classification. If you stutter because you inherited it from your generations or you acquired it from others through interaction, your stuttering is normal. My doctor was saying the other day that he didn't start stuttering from childhood and I said, 'You have a stuttering friend.' And he agreed. His two best friends stutter. They have been coming together from basic school. And the two of them are doctors too. So, their relationship has never been broken from childhood.

When I tell people that you can acquire stuttering, many don't agree with me. But it happens. It is rare but we have seen some cases. You know when you really love someone, whether a friend or a spouse, you naturally respect them. In the course of respect, you share each other's values, good or bad. So far you are comfortable with this person you can't see what other people may see as flaws. That is how some people can unconsciously develop brain connections for stuttering without actually having the gene for it.

Audience fear and anxiety also make some people stutter habitually. This is also normal stuttering. It happens when some people are shy and fainthearted. They just can't muster up the confidence or poise to control their organs. You see them start to repeat the same sound and words before getting it correctly. In time, the brain can create a connection for that behavior. And it will send signals regularly telling your body to do the same thing any time you face a similar situation.

The last two cases I mentioned are usually not as strong as genetically transferred stuttering. That's is the fact. And they don't happen all the time. Especially if a person stammers due to phobia and absence of confidence, the condition stops gradually as he gets bold and experienced. But stuttering due to heredity is generally more intense. But if it is observed in the kid early, it can be arrested easily as you will see in one of the sections of this book.

Fortunately though, all three cases mentioned are simple. This is because, the speech organs are always fine. They have no problem. You just need some push, some coordinations and something like that. That's all. If you make your brain active for it and discipline yourself along our instructions, you are going to use the process of habit-forming to overwrite stuttering in a short time.

The other types of stuttering are actually neurological. This guide will not handle that. The stuttering actions are actually influenced by some fundamental neuron issues. And you know what I mean. Nervous issues can arise at any time. A person can come with them from birth, and they can also happen after birth.

Look at some of these health conditions after birth that can affect the nerves. Severe Convulsions, ALS, Muscular Dystrophy, Stroke, Sclerosis, Parkinson's Disease.

And if the part of the brain that controls the muscles didn't develop well at conception, the person might also have difficulties controlling the muscles for speech. Some imbeciles are good example of this.

Stammer that originates from nervous problem can only be managed by therapists or caregivers. And if it's associated with illness like Parkinson's, the case gets bad overtime. And there's nothing the best therapist in the world can do about that.

That is why we actually say that nothing is wrong with you if your case falls within the normal stuttering. You are free.

3
PREPARING FOR THE PROGRAM

The things you need for this program are basically few. First, I will provide adequate empty pages for your use throughout the book. If you have the print edition, they are going to be very helpful. Otherwise, you are going to get your own journal to keep useful notes.

Another thing that you are going to need is something for recording yourself. There is no need to go for some complicated recording midget. If you have a mobile phone, you are good to go. The cheapest mobile these days has recorders. I will show you how you are going to use that to accelerate your progress.

You will also need a timetable. You will do a thorough study of this book and you have some activities to help you progress. And you have other things that you do everyday. Working with a timetable will help you to balance all that you do everyday with this program. You need to be regular and consistent with it for the best results.

I think this is all you need. If there are others they cannot be more than normal household items. Yes, like a full-length mirror. That should be available in your dressing room already. So, things like that, cheap and common home things.

Now, I will like us to go right to our main business from here. I want us to start with the major factor for smooth speeches and the correct actions to counter stuttering. I don't want us to start with what you do when you stutter, such as your behavior or posture or how you start to operate your hands and your legs. All those follow stuttering.

When we nip off the major issues, the appendages will die too. That is not to oversimplify the task of breaking those other habits. You are really also going to work to break them. But we will make it simple. It will make it easier to leave them when you learn what makes them happen.

Lets begin with your recorders.

NOTE:
Your timetable?
More

4

□□ STEP 1

HOW RECORDINGS CREATE A BASE FOR YOUR RECOVERY

We assume that by now you have your device ready for recording. Next, try to figure out two things. Identify a few subjects that are challenging for you to talk about with a measure of fluency. And figure out some situations that give your speeches a lot of trouble.

Next, try doing a speech on any of the hard subjects or situation. Have someone record you during the difficult speech.

Audiovisual is best for this activity. It doesn't only allow you hear and feel the performance of your voice. You will also be able to observe your movements, how you used your body parts or your behavior when you speak. We are going to talk about the effect of that later on.

But if you don't have a video recorder, don't worry. Just make only the audios.

These first few days, look for opportunities to speak in your most difficult situations and make sure they are recorded.

Then, store or keep your recordings in a safe place. You can save to Google drive or to other storage clouds that you have. And have a copy handy. This is what you are going to use as your reference base to contrast and to see how you are making progress each day.

Finally, spend some time to review your recordings. Do your review several times trying to identify the areas that you mostly have words collision. Try to observe your behavior during the time that you were speaking. Take note of the movements of your hands, legs, eyes, tongue or your lips.

But don't worry about how much of the unattractive behaviors you are able to isolate at this time. We are actually going to help you to identify more later on. Just note what you are able to see right now. Trying to do it now will help you to fix them more easily in your head when we begin to work on that area.

NOTE:
Your findings

5

□□ STEP 2

RELAXING YOUR SPEECH MUSCLES

The muscles of our body normally become tense when we are anxious or afraid. The same is true of the muscles for speaking. While a person that speaks fluently can still manage to get away with the situation, a stutterer experiences a high rate of word jam. This forms the basis for your understanding why he might often have difficulties with the first sound the word. Why, several thing can make him anxious when it comes to speaking.

He often fears that he is not going to talk right in front of a boss, when with a stranger, a person of the opposite sex or when he is required to justify his actions. And what he is afraid not to happen often happens in the end.

So, you are going to learn to relax all your muscles. And that is not going to be hard. The major factor in relaxing your muscles is your breathing.

Well, we are not actually trying to remind you that you need air to speak. That's not the point. The air you take in and out does more than that. Your ability to get calm is also factored into the amount of air that fills you and the way that air is sucked in.

Of course, most people do not need to think about this because they don't stutter. The human speech system and all that makes it up are so wonderful that we don't need some extra effort to hold some air in us in other to sustain our speech. They slowly release just the right amount of air that we need to speak. That is why most of us don't think about the relationship between our breath and our speech.

But for a stutterer or for someone who bops to speak or for a person who is training his voice for singing, coordinating the breath is a critical requirement.

So, you need breath control knowledge at the base level of this guide to serve a two-fold purpose in solving your speech problem. This will fix your voice quality. And second, it will keep down your nerves and muscles. Trust me, it is the fundamental requirement for those who want to solve stuttering, lisping and consonant omissions issues. If there is no nervous problem, this guide is going to correct your stammer and related issues in no time.

Let us now go into some details on how your breath can relax you muscles and fix the quality of your voice.

To relax your muscles, you need to watch out for either of two breathing types. They are lungs and chest breathing. Do you know how you breath when you are speaking? There is a little bit of trick here which I want to teach you.

Lungs breathing is the type of breathing that allows air to go right down to the bottom part of the lungs first before the upper part. And that really completely fills you out with air. So, there is enough to meet the body's need. This is the best type of breathing. It dilutes the tension that might be present in the muscles of your body. If your muscles are relaxed you are more likely to be yourself.

But chest breathing is a very shallow one. In this case only the upper part of the lungs are filled. First, it shortens the amount of air that you have in you to speak. So, you easily run out of air. Already, that is a problem to quality speech. This is how we breath involuntary when we feel threatened or so.

Unfortunately, this often happens to stutterer when he is speaking especially when he is afraid that he won't do it right.

Now you can see the biggest rock under the water. There is no need to tell you to try to figure out how you breathe when you are anxious about speaking. You do have chest breathing and that is always too shallow for a quality speech. If you have doubts try to observe. I will show you an experiment to do that later. But now, I want you to try something else first.

Just find some opportunity to be anxious about your speech. When you find one, do the following before you begin to speak. Take a deep breath, making sure your lower lungs are filled first. Keep taking it in until your whole lungs are filled. Then, start to talk, slowly and in a relaxed manner. Do you have any observation? Write down whatever you noticed.

NOTE:
What are the two breathing types?
What else did you learn?

But I assumed that when you took that deep breath and started speaking calmly, you got a more stabled voice. And that is the point I was making. Lungs breathing improves clarity and voice depth. Your muscles are relaxed enough for your sound pace and pitch to be very fine. The muscles of your voice box are not Squashed down by some pressure. They are free and ready to make thunderous sounds versus clipped ones. But if the breath is otherwise, you get some uncomfortably clipped and high-pitched sound. Even when a person doesn't stutter, this happens when the air inside is not adequate. You want to rush to pour out everything before you run out of air. If that can happen on a normal ground, you can imagine the devastation that's going to do to a stutterer's speech.

So, here is where we lay the foundation. Breath control is always our base architecture for stuttering resolution guide. We are now going to teach you how to regulate that consciously until your breath for speech are driven spontaneously. And as I said at the onset, all of this is going to take strong personal discipline from you. So, if you can give it, you'll be fine the soonest.

Later on, I'm going to help you to see exactly why you must start talking slowly after filling out your lungs. But I told you that there is a simple experiment to find out how you breathe. Let us do that experiment right now to see.

6

□□ STEP 3

YOUR BREATH ORIGIN

This simple test is going to help you make sure of how you breath. You will be able to confirm whether it is chest or lungs breathing.

Open one of your hands and rest it on the lower part of your belly. It should be in the area between your navel and the waistline. Stay calmly and monitor what you are feeling. You can be standing or sitting while you do this. If you are standing, you can push your hand down a little bit. If your lower belly goes up, pushing your hand outward, it is an indication of lungs breathing. Your hand is going to get some pressure in that lower area of your belly. That is to say that you are filling the lower part of your lungs before the air moves to the second phase and begin to fill your upper lungs.

But if you have chest breathing, you are not going to get that outward push against your hand. The air that is coming is not going down to the lower part of your lungs. This is because your lungs are squashed down, closing the airways and preventing the air from penetrating to the lower lungs. You will observe that it is only your shoulders that will be going up and down.

Breath coordination is the foundation phase of stuttering correction. Proper coordination has an amazing effect on your muscles. That is going to bring a lot of relief to all the muscles of your body. Your tongue, your jaws and all the muscles in your vocal cord's surroundings will calm down. That creates the right condition for your vocal cord to adjust without any hindrance.

Just test this out right now. Get your breath deep down to your bottom lungs before you fill the upper part. Allow several seconds to pass to let your muscles relax. Then, begin talking, starting out a little bit slower than the way you normally speak. Did you notice that your labor to say the first sound is reduced? And your speech is less jerky?

Did you know that when your muscles are relaxed you gain more confidence? You can see that you can't skip breath coordination step in this masterclass. Lungs breathing relaxes all your muscles. Relaxed muscles in turn leads to greater confidence. And good confidence enhances your flow of speech. So, you must learn and apply breath coordination as a foundation for the other lessons to sit.

There is also a simple experiment to test whether you have enough confidence. The way you use your body when you talk is a test of your confidence. When you are talking with your mouth and you are full of enthusiasm, your eyes talk too. Your hands, your face and all the other parts of your body make meaningful contributions too. They all join to convey your overall feelings to your listener.

But if you lose confidence, the way you are going to use your body will not follow the words coming from your mouth. Your hand might be fumbling with the edge of your shirt or it might be beating your legs as you labor to talk. You might be shuffling your feet on the floor. There are so many awkward things your body members can be doing that are not tidy. Once you start to display any of these mannerisms, you have stopped communicating. This is because your listener's attention will shift from what you are telling him and rest on you. He may start to feel sorry within him instead of hearing what you are saying.

To correct this, work on your breathing to relax your muscles. When your muscles are relaxed you become more poised. You can see that the value of breath coordination cannot be overemphasized. It is the base structure for all the other things that you will learn to break free from stuttering.

I guess that you have started to learn lungs breathing at this point. Start and avoid shallow breathing that comes from the chest. You can pick up a subject that is always difficult for you to talk about. Tell somebody to watch you and tell you about your physical bearing. He can tell you whether your gestures and body language were in line with your speech. You can also use a full-length mirror and observe by yourself. Check whether your neck or your shoulders are rigid. Check whether your hands are also talking or they are making some odd motions. You can discover a lot by yourself and use your breath to correct them.

Never become discouraged though, if you still feel your breath from your chest. The correction is not going to happen in one day. You must fix this in mind and try to do it every time. Try to remember often. That is why I told you before that all of this is going to take strong personal discipline from you. Your effort will yield result gradually and your speech will improve tremendously.

The following exercises will help you to practice and to master your breath until it becomes a natural thing to you. After the exercises, our next subject will be the techniques of speech.

ACTIVITIES

1. *GENERAL CHECK.* In order to remember to monitor your breathing, set reminders on your device. And set the device to a setting that won't cause distraction to others. Each time the reminder notifies you, cleverly rest a palm of your hand on your lower belly for a minute or so as you breathe normally. If you do this for a day or two, you are going to be able to confirm your breath.

   CHECK WHEN UNDER PRESSURE/ANXIOUS. If your verification shows that your breathing is okay after a day or two, then try to see how it is when you are speaking, anxious or under pressure. If it is shallow, you are going to work on that a little bit.
2. Effective immediately, take your time before you start talking. Take several seconds to breath deeply, in, out, in out. Then, start talking slowly every time. We will talk a little bit about that later on, why you will need to proceed slowly.
3. Effective immediately, begin to practice how to ease or

relax specific muscles that are important to your speech. Your shoulders, your neck, your tongue, your throat and your jaws are very vital among these. Of course, your tool to achieve this is taking your time to breathe well. To speed up the whole thing, set a goal of days as well as what you want to achieve within the set time period in breath coordination, relaxing specific muscles, taking your time a little bit before beginning to talk after a deep breath.

4. After some days, take up a difficult subject of discussion or intentionally face a situation that normally poses the biggest challenge to you. Record your performance. After that, compare your new recordings with your original recordings.

5. Rate your new recordings in terms of observed improvement.

NOTE:
Important things you discovered

STUTTERING

7

□□ STEP 4

SOUND, SPEECH AND THE SKILLS

In this lesson, we are going to have some fun. It is going to be like a game. I will challenge you to do something about sound. If you are able to do it, you become the winner. And remember that if you win, I win too, because we are in this together.

What you are going to do for me is give me all the complete sounds of every word you say. And you know what that is going to mean – talking very slowly. That is the only way all the sounds of each word can come out distinctly.

So, you are going to study what we have in this lesson very carefully to know why you are going to do this. And if you score everything, you will get 5 stars.

ACHIEVEMENT RATING
1. **Syllable Level:** Make all the sounds in each word you say come out clearly. Get □□
2. **Word Level:** Make every word you say very precise as if you are learning to talk all over again. Get □□
3. **Sentence Level:** Make every sentence of your speech slowly and patiently. Get □

Total: ☐☐☐☐☐
Set 5 of 5 stars as your goal.

Now let's see what we are trying to do. Because you cannot speak fluently doesn't mean that you don't understand that every spoken language has a structure. You are quite aware that a word is built from one or more smaller units called syllables. You also know very well that each of these small units that make up a word produces it's own separate sound.

But we know where you have a struggle as a stutterer. And we know why you face that challenge. We will help you to identify those factors.

Now, how should you treat a word since you know what it is made of? You need to start by going back to the drawing board and take a fresh look at those smaller bits that makes a word. Now you need to understand the damage those little elements can cause if they are ignored. Look at them again and assign to them their own sound in each word.

Lets break a few words down into their component syllables.
Component = com-po-nent
Syllable = sy-lla-ble
Understand = un-der-stand
Element = e-le-ment
Ignore = ig-nore
Identify = i-den-ti-fy
Unprofessional = un-pro-fe-ssion-nal
Forgive my unprofessional phonetic arrangement. But those examples may help you understand what we mean here. I recommend that you don't see words as one lump, but as Pieces. This is an area that you want to handle really nicely, effective immediately.

We know why you face this challenge. Two things cause this. The first one is rapid or very fast speech. Every stutterer faces this, speaks very fast any time he is fortunate and the speech flows. This time, he runs all the sounds together. The second occasion when the challenge comes is when he has an obstructed speech. This time, he swallows some sounds.

Taking a new look at the syllables of a word will help you to correct this eventually. You know, when you speak too fast, you slur or run words together. That can lead to lose of some valuable sounds or confused sounds that can change the meaning of an expression altogether. The same thing happens if sounds are muffled or swallowed. Some sounds get lost. Both slurred and muffled talk make it very easy to get your words obstructed or to interrupt yourself and begin to stutter.

Now we have identified why it is hard for you to assign sounds to the small bits that make up a word. This place is the point our game starts. **Syllable Level.** You must work hard and effective immediately, approach the words of your statements differently. And remember that we said that it is going to make you talk slowly. So, don't worry about slowness now. That is the first thing that we want to achieve now. And if you are able to make all the syllables of your words come out and maintain that new style, you will score two stars in the game. So, work hard to earn the two stars.

It will start to overwrite the former habits that is stored in your brain. Sometimes you are fluent, but at other times, your speech is jerky. That is what is originally stored in your brain. Now, as you slow down and take your time to make all the syllables count, you will begin to see a balance. You will see the north and the south coming to meet at a balanced point.

Remember that we have been able to prove earlier that the process of forming a new habit and breaking older ones is the same. And that the gene has only a little hold on you. The art of making your brain very active and the environment you expose yourself usually create new connections in your brain that control your new habits. And if your counter habits are stronger, the older fades out.

Next, let us trace the origin of your fast talking and let us see what we can gain from that knowledge. In two words, 'audience fear' is behind all of that. When under a situation that often challenges you, you are already afraid that you might stutter even before you begin to talk to the audience. By audience, we mean your listener. This can be one or more persons.

This audience fear began right from the time you started to stutter. It is mostly at home when you were still a child. Because you already realized that there is trouble with your speech, you fear that you would be jerky each time you want to talk to your parents, your siblings or other people around the home. But when you begin to talk and found that it started very fine, you are encouraged. So, you want to quickly rush out everything before they are obstructed.

That is how you begin to talk fast, from the time you started to stutter. A listener is waiting to hear what you have to say. You are afraid of him because you are not sure the words would come out straight. But the words finally come out smoothly. So, you are in a rush to pour out everything at once. Eventually the brain picks up the pattern. It grows into you and becomes a part of your life.

Now let us take out our profit from this thing we just figured out. We are going to start by isolating the players in this problem. 1. An impatient audience (one or more person). 2. Fear of disappointment and 3. A reality, that is a very rapid speech. Trust me, every stutterer talks very fast whenever it is flowing for them. So, what is the solution?

Win the second leg of our game and correct this problem. **Word Level.**

First, make your impatient audience wait. Stop thinking that they are in a hurry to hear you out. Learn to behave like Narcissus who fell in love with a reflection of himself in a pool of water. Adore yourself in front of your listeners. Lift yourself above your audience no matter how impatient it might seem to be. You are a free moral agent. You have every right reserved for you. No one else's presence should rightfully force you to fear or try to do something beyond your capacity. This attitude is going to kill your fear too.

As a stutterer, talking too fast hurts than heal your effort. We are going to detail that a little bit later on.

Learning this new attitude will help you to avoid thinking that someone's presence is commanding you to act out of fear. You are a god by yourself. Even the Christian Holy book says so in a few places including John 10:34. Each one of us is unique. So, always take your time, breath very deeply to your bottom belly for a few seconds to relax your nerves. And slowly, start to say something, going at a pace that is more comfortable for you to handle. Endeavor to make all the sounds of each word clear and precise.

Rise above your audience, kill every fear, create a new reality (slow talking) and earn two more stars.

Admittedly, you have been talking very fast all your life. But trust me, your brain is going to build new connections to operate your new habit, your new reality. This will fade out the older habit and make you smile.

All of this will take patience from you for things to get natural again. A few changes will happen that are going to affect your speech at the beginning. Some of them might even make you feel ashamed because somebody might think that you are learning to talk. But don't worry. That's his own business. As I said before, that is the aim of this particular lesson. And if we are able to get that result, then, we have hit the mark.

So, remember! Approach every word of your statement as a lump that is built from smaller pieces. Assign a sound to every syllable. Call every word you say precisely. Breathe deeply and always take a little bit of time before you start to talk. And always star slowly.

Now earn the last point, one star. **Sentence Level.** Make a few sentences. Observe whether you were able to sound the words of the sentences more precisely. And you will receive one more star.

An old habits can never die for you in 24 one day. So, practice is very essential to get absorbed in your new realities and to wipe out the older one. Regular effort will help your tongue and your jaws to start adjusting to normal movement. Keep practicing. And if you are able to bring the speed of your speech near it's minimum, that is evidence that we have made progress. And the frequency of sound accidents that make you stammer will be reduced too. And that gives you 5 of 5 stars. And have no fear or shame about slowness. You will start to talk normally again after some time. By that time, you will have completely recovered from stuttering. You will win because a winner is what I want to be all the time.

ACTIVITIES

1. The words below are broken down to their smaller units. Practice pronouncing each of them, saying the separate sound of each of the little units.
   O-ppor-tu-ni-ty
   Per-for-mance
   Work-sheet
   Im-prove-ment
   A-cci-dent
   Mi-ni-mum
   Ob-jec-tive
   Pro-gress
   E-ssen-tial
2. Write down your own words that you would like to break

down and practice their syllables. Try to observe how careful you were to make sure all the sounds come out.

3. Make every opportunity you have to talk with someone beneficial. Watch yourself and see how slow and relaxed you could be at every occasion.

   If there is no one to talk to, try talking in front of a full-length mirror, to yourself. Then, try to see how relaxed you could be.

4. After practicing for a day or two, make a video. Check how much you still slur or muffle words. Watch for how clear you now sound out syllables, full words and the words in your sentences.

Continue to practice this everyday any time. Your active brain is going to overwrite the odd habits just after a few days. Keep repeating the activities. Your talk will get smoother.

NOTE:
What do you want to remember?

STUTTERING

8

□□ STEP 5

OTHER ENEMIES OF PROGRESS

I'm sure that you are taking every opportunity to practice the things we have learned so far. When you compare your recordings did you see that you are getting nearer to winning? Expectedly, your performance in the newer videos should be quite better than the older recordings.

Now, there are other major hindrances to the smooth flow of your speech. We are going to figure them out and also consider how to go forward and continue to improve.

When a stutterer's speech begins to get jerky, he starts to welcome one or all of these three enemies. The first one is ONE WORD IN A MILLION HOURS. The second is REGRESSION. And the third one is NOISE. These three are probably the biggest problems that you have with jerky speeches.

If you have mastered what we already taught you before now, you can completely solve your stutter problem. But if you do not conquer these three enemies, your speeches will still be jerky even though you don't stutter anymore. Now let's see why.

Bear in mind that it is not only a stutterer that suffers interruptive sound accident in speeches. But the occurrence is only more often in his case. After that, you can still continue to flow if you don't do any of the three things above. Let us start with the first one, 'One word in a million hours.'

When an interruptive sound accident happens, a stutterer will keep struggling to complete the statement by all means. He hangs his breath in his chest and keep pushing because he thinks that an impatient listener is waiting for him to finish the statement. Keep in mind that the harder you push, the stronger the wall gets. If you refuse to breathe, you can't say the first sound of that challenging word in a million hours, so to speak.

So, when sound from your mouth hit the wall, stop at once. Don't try harder. Take your time. Breathe, relax and start to talk again at a slow pace that you can maintain. Don't worry about how long you paused. It makes your statements neat. And if you continue to practice this, your brain will pick it up. You will get better fluency in no time.

The bottom line: whenever you are interrupted by stuttering, stop at once. Don't push further.

'Regression' is the second impediment to a smooth speech. After stuttering, you want to resume your statement. The easiest thing to do is to go back to the beginning of the sentence to start. That's wrong. It is best to resume from exactly the word where you had a problem. It doesn't make others understand you better if you go back. But if you start from where it was broken, you get a very nice talk because your words linked properly. Don't also worry about the length of waiting. Don't start to wriggle or fumble around. Just breath for a few seconds and continue.

'Noise' is the number three enemy of fluency. When your speech is interrupted by stuttering, do not improvise some sound to fill the gap until you recover. That's what happens to even some public speakers. You can compare those who fill gaps with noise versus those who do not. You will find some appealing magic in the presentations of those who do not insert noise.

Some examples of noise include: 'em', 'uuuh', 'you know', 'so' 'you see', 'ar, and stuff like that. You must have listened to some interviews where those being interviewed showed one of those mannerisms. Sometimes, 'you now' is inserted after every statement. So, half of the answers given by the interviewed is 'you know' and the other half is actually the answers given.

But why do most people include these undesirable sounds in

their speech? When they have a pause and need a moment to process their thought about what to say next, they try to fill the moment with something.

But we want you to have it in mind that they have nothing to add to the objective of your speech. They contribute no additional meaning. That is why they are called semantic noise. And noise is actually what they are.

Before we get to the activities part of this section, you may make a recording of both situations right now to prove the truthfulness of this.

So, when stammering stops your talk abruptly, do as we said before when we talked about one word in a million hours. Just pause. Don't insert any sound to fill the gap. And don't push. No matter how long the pause, leave it blank. Semantic noise only litters your speech.

So, take special note of these three enemies of progress to fluency. Avoid pushing needlessly to say one word in a million hours. Stop at once. Take a breath and and continue again, slowly. Avoid regression, going back and for when stammer cuts you short. Continue exactly from the last word that gave you a little bit of problem. And finally, don't improvise some sound to fill a pause gap. Leave the space blank, no matter how long the pause.

Are you enthusiastic about these things that you are learning? If you are, start to practice immediately. You have opportunities. Start using them at once. You must have been happy now by the changes you are seeing in yourself. Find some friendly faces among your friends, family, schoolmates and other acquaintances. Strike a conversation and try to apply the tips that you learned. You can also talk in front of a mirror and use these techniques. The more you use them, the more they become part of you and the sooner you are going to succeed in overcoming stuttering.

ACTIVITIES

Prepare to give a lengthy talk on one of your difficult subjects. You can present it to a physical audience or to your reflection in a mirror. If you stutter when you read from a book, choose your topic from a book. If not, present your topic from your head using your normal everyday style of speech.

1. Observe how quickly you are able to stop when your

statement is obstructed. Repeat it several times and note your improvements. Did you react faster each time you repeat?

2. Have you stopped going back to the beginning of a sentence?

3. Have you tried not to insert some noise to fill a pause gap? Are you able to endure a pause than before? What if the pause is taking longer and becoming embarrassed? Can you still leave the space blank?

4. After practicing for a day or two, make new recordings. Then, compare the cleanness of your speech with your older recordings. Does it prove that the situation is getting better? Are you walking closer to overcoming stuttering each day?

5. Commendation will give you more strength to do more. So, don't look at only flaws and areas that you still need to work hard. Learn to also tell yourself 'well done' in the areas that you have started to do well.

NOTE:
Points I need to work on

9

▢▢ STEP 6

GESTURE, FACIAL EXPRESSIONS AND BODY LANGUAGE

We have said before that the voice is only a small factor when it comes to passing information effectively from us to other people. To help others capture the overall intent of our expressions, our hands speak, and so are our face and the other parts of the body. From simple talks with family members and neighbors to the more professional public presentations, all of our body contribute to the success of our communication.

Therefore, in order not to lose valuable information, our body and our voice must speak in agreement. Our voice should not be saying one thing and the other body members saying something else. If you are talking to someone and your eyes begin to shoot out of their sockets how would your listener feel about that? He would begin to sympathize with you rather than listen to you. Under that situation, much of the things you said would just be given to the wind.

So, you can see that your voice is not just everything in talking. That is why after giving you the gist earlier, I said that we would still talk about it in some details.

When you have an opportunity to talk to someone, or someone has the opportunity to listen to you, what you have in mind to say is important to both of you. But if your voice and your body fail to agree with each other, a lot of that information would be lost.

For instance. You are talking to someone. One of your hands is going in and out of your pocket just because you don't have enough confidence. Or you shuffle your feet on the floor. Or you begin to look at the floor to avoid eye contact. You will get your audience to say, 'Oh my God! What makes this guy thinks he is so small?' And if you beat yourself as you talk or your tongue sticks out or your eyes bulge from the sockets, your audience gets the impression that you are laboring. He would start to feel pity for you. He won't hear much of the things that you said.

So watch yourself when you are talking. If you feel nervous, try relaxing your muscles. Take a breathe, a deep one. Relax your neck and your jaws. Stop rushing yourself, stop pushing. Start talking slowly and calmly.

Aren't you glad to identify these hidden fact that might be affecting your speech? Practice how to talk harmoniously with all of your body. You will see how it works like magic. Your voice is going to gain a lot from this.

ACTIVITIES

1. Tell someone to assess you for slovenly speech. He should tell you if your appearance is sloppy. You can tell him something specific to watch for. If he says there is evidence of any odd gesture, set aside time on your timetable to practice and to correct it immediately.

2. After practicing good gestures and postures for a day or two, make some video recordings. Compare your new videos with the older ones. If you find some improvements, tell yourself 'well done,' and continue until no trace of awkward movements remain when you speak.

NOTE:
Odd body language I need to correct
Something else that I identified

10

☐☐ STEP 7

BUILDING ON YOUR PERSONAL EFFORTS

Trust me, this is the biggest secret. If you get what it take to do it, your miracle would take no longer than three weeks to happen. How are you going to build on the foundation that you have personally laid?

Other people can complement your personal effort. If there are some loved ones who might be willing to help, that also can fast-track your recovery. By this I do not mean stutterers communities. I don't like communities at all because they discourage you from trying to recover. I have joined several before, but they don't want you to talk about recovery. All they do is tell you how to handle your day to day challenges in your situation. Some groups removed me and I left others by myself because they don't want to hear that you say there is a solution.

I have the simple solution so, I don't like those foundations. I'm happy because those who have passed through my masterclasses are happy too. I love them and we will continue to rejoice together even though I will never meet some of them in person.

This is how good friends and family members can help you. You will need to pause. Keep that in mind. That is the most difficult of everything that you are required to do and it is the key thing too. You must pause instantly whenever stuttering interrupts your statement. A friend can give you alert to pause. When you pause, you can breathe and resume slowly. You and the person can agree on what sign to give you. I often recommend raising a hand. If he raises a hand or lift a thumb, nobody around would know what's happening.

You can also share some of the things you have learned with him. Tell him some of the things you must do and others that you need to avoid.

If you can get this help, trust me, in two or three weeks, you are a different person entirely when it comes to talking smoothly.

NOTE:
My friend helps me about ….

11

PARENTS, NIP IT IN THE BUD

Stuttering starts mostly from childhood. If you are a parent, you can detect it as soon as it starts. If you observe very well, stuttering is not really the inability to say a word or a sentence. It is actually connected with the first sound of a word. It is the struggle to say that first sound of a word. It doesn't matter where it happened. It could be at the beginning of a statement and it could be within or at the end.

If you child is learning to talk and he wants to say daddy. He says da-da-da-da-da, or he is trying to say mommy. He says mo-mo-mo-mo, or he is doubling on words, that is saying one word twice every time, do not just watch to see. Start to show him your love and begin to help him immediately. Don't relax especially if there is stuttering trait in your family.

Well, we all know that most parents get away with ignoring the condition in their stuttering kids. This is because most people who stutter as kids give it up as they grow. But which child will give it up? Nobody knows. So, it's better to help the kids when he is tender than to let stuttering set him up for trouble in the future.

And keep in mind that it is not difficult at all to help a stuttering kid. All you need do is to tell him to stop. Then, figure out the word he is trying to say. Help him to say the word. After saying it, tell him to say the word now. If he stammers again or say the word twice, stop him again. Repeat the word to him again. Then, tell him to say it again once. Keep repeating this process every time he starts to stutter. And within a week or two, his brain will pick it up. Their brain is like a white paper sheet. Anything that enters, sticks.

That's what I did to help all my kids, five of them. They all showed that tendency to stutter. I realize they got the gene for stammer from me. But my wife and I helped each one of them as they come. And it was fun. They're all growing up. And if we tell them that they started the journey when they were much younger, they argue with us every time.

You can do the same for your child if their early speech is tending towards that direction.

NOTE:
I am doing these things for my stuttering child

12

LISPING AND CONSONANT OMISSION

Some people don't stutter, but they don't enunciate clearly. It is either because they lisp or because they omit certain consonants when they enunciate some words.

A person who lisps pronounces 'S' and 'Z' sounds as /θ/, which is a voiceless dental fricative form of 'th' sound. Somebody could be 'Thomebody,' and Zebra could come out as 'Thebra.'

Similarly, a person with consonant omission is short of certain consonants in his tongue, so to speak. So, when he speaks, he improvised the missing letters, with other similar sounds. 'L' and 'R' sounds are the most commonly lost consonants. And 'V' is in some rare cases. In this case, London could be expressed as 'Yondon,' Road as 'Yoad' or 'Load,' and Venus as 'Fenus.'

The above examples do not apply to tonal languages such as Chinese, which has a different language structure. Lisping and consonant omission could convey a confusing idea or a totally change of meaning to the audience.

Lisping is a little bit harder to correct because it's going to be a little tedious for the memory to watch for 'S' and 'Z' every time you are talking. So, we have some practical activities to save you all the nerve wreck.

ACTIVITIES

1. LISPING: Select a lengthy passage from any of your favorite books. Use a pencil with deep lead to underline the 'S' and 'Z' sounds of the words in the passage. Use the passage to practice by reading it out aloud. Each time you are about to pronounce the sound of those marked letters, pull your tongue away from your teeth. What did you observe?

   Pronounce the word 'Simple' with your tongue touching your teeth. Take note of the sound you got. Pronounce the same word again with your tongue moved back from your teeth. Did you see any difference? So, it's just fun practicing these things. Practice and play, that's all.

   To make it even easier, try this reading skill. Allow your eyes to pick word groupings rather than seeing each word in isolation. Seeing word groupings makes it easier for you to spot 'S' or 'Z' on time and take the necessary action before enunciating their sounds inside a word.

2. CONSONANT OMISSION: Write down the consonants that you have trouble with. They are likely 'L', 'R' and 'V,' depending on your language structure. Have some fun, playing with them, that's all.

   To gain 'L', practice pushing the tip of your tongue under your upper teeth. Add a little bit of voice to make 'L' function as a voiced dental fricative. (Li li li li li li li li)

   For 'R' sound, the tip of the tongue will be pulled away from under the upper teeth. As the distance increases, the sound gradually changes from li li li li li ri ri ri ri ri ri. Your tongue will start rolling. But that little added voice needs to remain as your pull the tongue under your palate. Let 'R' in this practice also function as a voiced dental fricative. With continuous practice, your tongue will soon begin to reverberate against your palate which is called tongue rolling.

   Finally 'V' and 'F' sounds are obtained in a common way. This is by allowing your lower lip and your upper teeth to touch. But to get the sound of 'V' and 'F' separately, identify their dental fricatives. 'V' is voiced, while 'F' is voiceless.

3. After practicing for a day or two, make some recordings and compare them with your older ones. Tell yourself 'well done' for the progress you have made.

NOTE:
Areas I'm affected and my plan to fix them

13
FINAL WORD

Keep practicing and keep noting down areas you need to give more attention. And don't procrastinate. Make definite arrangements to fix them. Keep making new recordings too, to track your progress.

In the end, you will find that stuttering is easy to overcome. It is not a destiny that you must live with as our communities would tell you. And it's not indelible just because it is in the gene. Rather, your active brain will create new synapses for your new pattern of speech. And the more consistent you are with your practice sessions, the earlier you are going to see yourself free from the grips of stuttering.

Send your joys, your queries and your feedback to readingplx@gmail.com. All the best of fortune.

GRATITUDE

Thanks for studying this book. If you don'tmind, kindly give us a little bit
more of your time to rate the book. I'm grateful.
ARLO MASON

www.ingramcontent.com/pod-product-compliance
Lightning Source LLC
Chambersburg PA
CBHW012310240726
48656CB00008B/2635